STRESS IN MEDICINE

stress in medicine

Lessons Learned Through My Years as a Surgeon, from Med School to Residency, and Beyond

DR. NINA AHUJA, MD

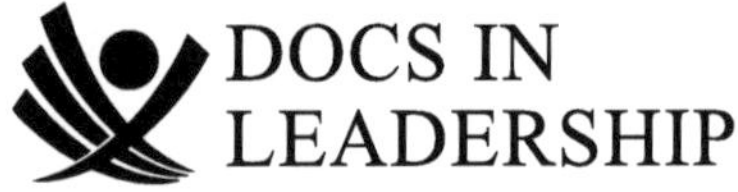

STRESS IN MEDICINE

Lessons Learned Through My Years as a Surgeon, from Med School to Residency, and Beyond

ISBN   978-1-5445-1745-2 *Hardcover*

978-1-5445-1743-8 *Paperback*

978-1-5445-1744-5 *Ebook*

Contents

Introduction 9

PART 1: NAVIGATING MEDICINE

1. A Unique Journey 21
   Becoming a physician is a unique journey that cannot be understood unless you've been through it.

2. The Nature of Stress 31
   Before you learn how to manage stress effectively, you first need to understand your own responses to stress and how they manifest themselves in your world.

3. The Nature of Uncertainty 45
   The root of stress is uncertainty. Reframing uncertainty as opportunities for growth helps increase your comfort with the unknown.

PART 2: UNDERSTANDING ADMIT

4. Adapting to New Ways 59
   New circumstances take time to get used to. Change your mindset to allow yourself to accept something new.

5. **Doing the Work**.. 73
*When you are pulled in all directions and feeling
overwhelmed, stressors beyond patient care are common.*

6. **Measuring Success**.................................... 83
*Defining internal measures of success helps keep
outcomes of external measures in perspective.*

7. **Introspection** 91
*Many new experiences and challenges will surely come
your way. Mindfulness and active reflection are essential.*

8. **Transformation** 103
*With the many influences around you and those that
shaped you, what kind of physician will you be?*

PART 3: SUPPORT

9. **The Importance of Support** 115
*Highs and lows are a normal part of medicine and life in
general. Having social support is essential for well-being.*

Conclusion 129

About the Author.................................... 133

Introduction

> *"Where the art of medicine is loved, there is also a love of humanity."*
>
> —HIPPOCRATES

I still remember the thrill of putting my own stethoscope around my neck for the first time. No longer was it the motivating prop I envisioned myself wearing when I thought of becoming a doctor. Now it was a diagnostic tool I would use to assess patients as a real-life MD. After years of hard work, dedication, commitment, and sacrifice, I had finally made it. I received and accepted an offer of admission to medical school, and I walked the halls of a teaching hospital with a feeling of excitement and curiosity. I peeked into patient rooms during my orientation of the clinical teaching unit, keen to get a glimpse into the world of working with patients. I felt joy and satisfaction that I was well on my way to fulfilling my dream of becoming a physician. A new phase of adventure would soon begin, and I couldn't wait to get started. I was prepared for more hard work and the responsibility that would come with my every decision directly impacting patients' lives. Not knowing exactly what to expect, I felt somewhat nervous. However, my commitment to learning to care for patients as best as I could overwhelmed any feelings of apprehension I felt at the time. Before I knew it, my years in medical school passed, followed by residency in ophthalmology, and I became a Royal College of Physicians and Surgeons of Canada certified specialist.

Through my years of training and as my surgical practice progressed, I gained insight into the world of medicine as I managed patients on the front line in teaching hospitals, community hospitals, private offices, and on a charitable mission. I experienced moments of profound joy and satisfaction, and moments of deep sadness and disappointment. As my practice grew, so did my responsibilities. I had more patients to care for, but with fewer resources available as constraints within the health system increased. Government funding for surgical cases became restricted. Hospital budget cuts resulted in fewer nurses in the OR and less administrative support in clinics, leaving those who remained feeling overwhelmed and overworked. My work as a physician was changing as well because of increasing bureaucracy, added administrative burden, and greater integration of digital technology in each patient interaction. With increasing reliance on electronic medical records, for example, there was more interaction with computer screens during an assessment than direct engagement and eye contact with my patients. While I liked the experience of progress and change, it was negatively impacting how I preferred to relate to my patients, and the sense of fulfilment from my work was slowly diminishing. My stress began to build.

While my professional world around me continually changed, my personal life continued to evolve as well. Married during residency, the relationship failed three years later due to a patriarchal undercurrent that became intolerable. I became hesitant to share stories about my interests and my work, and I began to feel disconnected from who I was. The first few years after the divorce focussed on self-reflection, rebuilding, and growth with wonderful support from my family and friends, after which a social event brought a new man into my life. He was a single dad with two young daughters and a joyful sense of humor. We took time to get to know one another, and I felt increasingly reassured as his actions aligned with mutual respect and equality. Helping the little one learn how to read, listening to the eldest share stories from school, and enjoying weekly pizza and movie nights became part of my world. Four years later we married, I officially became a stepmom, and my husband and I worked together to strengthen the bonds of our new blended family.

As my professional interests continued to evolve over the years, my involvement in academic work, committee work, leadership, and administration also increased. This helped restore my sense of fulfilment that was otherwise beginning to weigh on me. I juggled family commitments along with my work and was grateful to be living a full life. Between early morning meetings, never-ending paperwork, and rearranging schedules to bring the children to school when I could, I routinely wished each week had just one more day. I loved my family, I loved my work, and I was fully committed to both. However, I often felt my head and heart strings pulled in multiple directions.

When COVID-19 happened, my usual daily routine was suddenly forced to stop. Provincially mandated closures of all elective medical and surgical activities impacted my practice significantly, especially given the close proximity of patients during eye exams requiring slit lamp microscopes. While my leadership activities continued, the non-urgent closures offered an opportunity for personal and professional reflection. I had time to thoughtfully consider my journey, where I was, how I got there, and how I wished to proceed moving forward.

Through this period, my academic leadership role brought my awareness to the stresses being faced by faculty, medical students, and residents. We were all impacted in various ways; however, final-year students were especially concerned about impending certification exams and how their applications to residency programs and fellowships would be impacted. These were unprecedented worries for them on top of the usual stresses associated with being a medical student or resident. I began reading various blog posts expressing heartfelt concerns and frustrations, many of which deeply resonated with me and my days during medical school and residency. While beautifully written and openly expressive, these posts were often written anonymously.

As I reflected on the anonymity and my own professional and personal struggles over the years, I realized that I myself had often hesitated to openly share challenges with my colleagues. I had adopted and accepted the culture of silence within medicine in a manner that was entirely subconscious. It was rare that colleagues shared their inner struggles with me, so it never occurred to me to share with them.

With frustration, pessimism, and the risk of burnout in our profession near an all-time high, I realized that something had to change. We were all in the same profession; we all understood our unique context and could offer support to one another in meaningful ways. I had to challenge our culture of silence and decided to share stories from my own journey in medicine. I coined a framework called **ADMIT** to bring together strategies that have helped me manage my stress, advocate for my own health, and in turn care for patients more effectively. My hope is that this book will help you do the same.

The ADMIT framework is intended to help anyone dealing with the unique stresses, pressures, and joys of the medical profession. It can be applied in all contexts professionally and personally and offers an organized approach to assessing stress in relation to five phases of experience. You will learn what these five phases are and the factors that contribute to stress within each. My goal is for this framework to be top of mind, so that when you encounter challenging situations you can automatically self-assess and apply key takeaways to help you manage your stress effectively.

After completing residency at the University of Ottawa nearly two decades ago, I began my surgical practice in Hamilton, Ontario, Canada. I was appointed to a faculty position and was a key contributor in establishing the residency program for ophthalmology at McMaster University. There I developed a surgical teaching curriculum for cataract surgery that earned our program a reputation of excellence. As owner of my own private practice, I have also held numerous senior leadership roles at both academic and hospital organizations, including Academic Division Head, Medical Staff Association President, and member of the Board of Directors. I am certified in EQ-i 2.0® Emotional Intelligence assessment, and I founded *Docs in Leadership*, an organization to promote and provide emotionally intelligent leadership education to physicians and fellow health professionals.

Having been actively involved in medical education

for over 15 years, I have mentored residents, medical students, and early career surgeons through their training and onto independent practice, winning numerous awards for excellence in surgical teaching and contributions to medical education. My years of experience in various contexts have given me a unique and in-depth understanding of the challenges and stresses faced by medical students, residents, physicians, and surgeons.

This book is part memoir, part self-improvement: a thoughtful collection of reflections and lessons that I have learned over the course of my medical career. While it draws from theories on emotional intelligence, positive psychology, adult developmental theory, and others, this book is not an academic work but is intended to be a helpful companion for medical professionals.

We'll start by laying the groundwork for ADMIT: our first step is to understand and appreciate the unique journey that is medicine.

PART 1

Navigating Medicine

Memories of medical school, clinical clerkship, residency, and early practice. Smelling the unforgettable odours of embalming chemicals in the anatomy lab and falling asleep beside a preserved human brain. Hearing the haunting cries of parents after breaking the news that their beloved child has died and asking myself if anything more could have been done. Informing someone that they have a terminal illness and trying to console them in their sadness. Seeing past the jarring image of a nail sticking out of an eye, as I planned my technique for emergency surgery to remove it.

When one decides to pursue medicine, it is generally from a place of wanting to help others and make a tangible difference in their lives. The journey is filled with highs and lows. Medical school and residency are both intense experiences that bring professional and personal growth in unexpected ways. Many would say, aren't all professions like that? Surely, they are. But medicine is a unique and meaningful journey because these experiences and growth happen in circumstances that deal with the most vulnerable states of being human. I could not have imagined that in my second year of residency in ophthalmology, I would be sitting at the main operating microscope with my supervisor observing, as I removed shards of glass from a 10-year-old's eyes for two hours, following a motor vehicle accident that had shattered the windshield. It was my first time operating unassisted in an ocular trauma case. I could hear my heart beating as I maintained a steady hand, knowing that the slightest slip could cause more damage.

In medicine, life, death, and the quality of both are quite literally in your hands every day. In this section, we'll explore the challenges and stresses inherent in our profession, to lay the groundwork for my ADMIT framework and how it can help you navigate the unique world of medicine.

CHAPTER 1

A Unique Journey

"The purpose of a doctor or any human in general should not be to simply delay the death of the patient, but to increase the person's quality of life."

—PATCH ADAMS, MD

As physicians, we are privileged to have uniquely personal interactions with patients who are usually complete strangers. In my third month of medical school while on horizontal elective, my preceptor talked me through delivering a baby independently. I remember holding the newborn in awe, witnessing the heartwarming joy of the new parents, unable to move as I tried to process what had just happened. I was so moved by the experience of helping a new life enter the world that it took me several moments to hear my preceptor's voice repeatedly saying, "Nina, you can put the baby down—we need to cut the umbilical cord."

Patients carry an implicit trust in our capabilities and intentions as physicians. We're granted open access to engage and probe well beyond superficial niceties, all to help us understand how to best apply our knowledge and expertise to improve their conditions. We seek answers to intimate questions on a daily basis:

Does the patient have suicidal thoughts, and if so, do they have a plan?

Are they sexually promiscuous and at risk for sexually transmitted diseases that could explain their condition?

Did they really rupture their eye because they accidentally rolled out of bed and hit the corner of their nightstand, or was it the result of domestic abuse?

Do they have medical benefits for what health insurance doesn't cover, and if not, can they pay for the medication they need?

When I was a student physician, it took me a while to get used to asking patients details about themselves.

These sorts of questions seemed so personal and out of bounds with anyone I generally interacted with, especially strangers. My supervisor eventually had to make the point that asking these questions was an essential part of my job. I was *expected* to ask deeper questions. It was *necessary* to ask deeper questions. It was my *responsibility* to ask deeper questions to help complete the picture of a presenting complaint so I could review the case and formulate an appropriate treatment plan for my patients. All of this took time for me to internalize, but when I did, I realized that these unique rules of engagement between patients and physicians form the basis of meaningful care.

LEARNING DIFFERENTLY

While learning to interact with patients in a more inquisitive manner, I was also initially overwhelmed by the sheer *volume* of knowledge and skills I needed to learn, and in ways that were different than what I was used to. Didactic lectures were the norm in my undergraduate studies, so the shift to self-directed, problem-based, experiential learning at my medical school was significant and took longer for me to adapt to than I expected. Formal exams were now a thing of the past, so I had fewer quantitative measures to help me track my progress. I felt a heightened sense of personal responsibility to ensure that I would learn all that I needed to know. What lingered was a constant feeling of uncertainty that made the weight of that responsibility even heavier. I found myself second-guessing each diagnosis and triple-checking every order I wrote, recognizing that even the smallest error could have life-altering consequences for my patients.

Whether we realize or not, the 90,000 physicians, 10,000 residents, and 8,000 medical students across Canada alone are all challenged in ways that transform us from within. While each day is filled with knowledge-based transactions, the interactions we have with our patients and their families can't help but change us. I still remember the sweet elderly lady who had successful cataract surgery and cried with her daughter when she was able to see her family photo for the first time in years. Her response was humbling and reminded me of the impact of my work; it also made me realize how I took my own health and well-being for granted. Then there was the patient who rudely expressed her displeasure when her appointment was delayed, due to an urgent on-call assessment for a patient who, like me, happened to be of East Indian heritage. When this patient in the waiting room commented, "I guess you need to be brown to be seen around here," how could I have not felt appalled by the disrespect, discrimination, and entitlement?

DEVASTATING INJURIES

Then there were those interactions that struck me profoundly in other ways. On more than one occasion, I have been called to the neonatal intensive care unit to assess an intubated infant with head injury and multiple fractures. The purpose of these consults is to assess for the presence of retinal hemorrhages to confirm or counter the presumed diagnosis of non-accidental head trauma, otherwise known as shaken baby syndrome.

This is never an easy task, and one particular instance stands out in my mind. As I approached the crib, I saw a tiny two-month-old baby boy with soft tendrils of blond hair lying on his back completely still—his arms and legs extended, his head tilted slightly to one side. I noticed the plastic tubing in his nose that was helping him breathe, and wires that led to monitors beeping softly to the rhythm of the baby's heartbeat. His head looked much larger than usual, as would be expected with cerebral edema. I noticed a tiny splint supporting a fracture on his right arm. I suddenly found myself aware of the baby's ten little fingers and ten little toes, and a wave of sadness and compassion came over me. My thoughts turned to the person suspected of inflicting this injury. How could the person do this? What were the circumstances and mindset? Would the baby return home to a place of safety? Did this person realize the likelihood of everlasting impact on this defenseless child?

Despite the troubling thoughts that went through my mind, I carried out my assessment objectively as always. With dilating and topical anesthetic drops administered, I placed a lid speculum on the baby's right eye to keep it open for the exam. I checked my indirect ophthalmoscope headset to ensure that it was securely in place, then adjusted its light intensity to a brightness that would allow a clear view. I gently turned the baby's head towards me and used my hand-held lens and scleral depressor to focus the light and look for signs of trauma in the eye. The baby seemed to flinch slightly, and I was keenly aware of how uncomfortable the bright light could be. I gently removed the speculum and repeated the process on the left eye. I felt another wave of sadness and compassion come over me, as I saw clear evidence in both eyes that the baby had likely been abused. After completing my consult notes, I slowly drove home and quietly reflected.

A COMPLEX EXPERIENCE

The journey of medicine is emotionally intense, exhilarating, rewarding, and one that cannot be understood unless you have been through it firsthand. There are moments of joy so powerful that you feel privileged for your work. There are moments so challenging and stressful that you feel sadness that can be overwhelming and difficult to express.

Through most of my journey in medicine, I have rarely heard anyone talk about how extraordinary these situations are—we all seem to carry on, "business as usual." Much of our work requires us to internalize our emotions so that we can calmly and objectively care for patients. The risk is that our emotional processing may become blunted and begin to impact us in ways we may not expect.

It is essential to remind ourselves that we are all colleagues who face similar situations in our own contexts. Sharing our experiences and perspectives with one another will not only promote our well-being for ourselves, our families, our patients, and our teams, but also serve to challenge the culture of silence in medicine. The ADMIT framework offers a common approach to understanding and managing stress in ways that can be applied personally and professionally.

In the next chapter, we will explore the true nature of stress.

KEY TAKEAWAYS

- Becoming a physician is a unique journey that cannot be understood unless you've been through it yourself.

- The current culture of silence in medicine discourages one from acknowledging and sharing stressful experiences for fear of being judged negatively in some way.

- The ADMIT framework provides an approach to understanding sources of stress and learning to manage contributing factors effectively.

REFLECTION POINTS

(Take time for yourself to consider your answers and keep them in mind as you progress through the book.)

- Why did you want to be a doctor?

- How have your expectations been met, or not, so far in your career?
- What professional experiences have profoundly impacted you personally?

CHAPTER 2

===

The Nature
of Stress

"You can't control everything—your hair was put on your head to remind you of that!"

—UNKNOWN

As you move through life and face challenges along the way, your responses to stress vary and can even be rather quirky. When I first learned that I was accepted into McMaster medical school, I was ecstatic. Hours of filling out applications and watching the popular television show *ER* for motivation (even with its inaccuracies!) were all worth it as I anticipated starting the academic year. When September drew near and I began preparing for my move to Hamilton, I booked my usual return-to-school appointment with my hairdresser. I had worn my hair just above my shoulders through most of high school and undergrad (see Exhibit A).

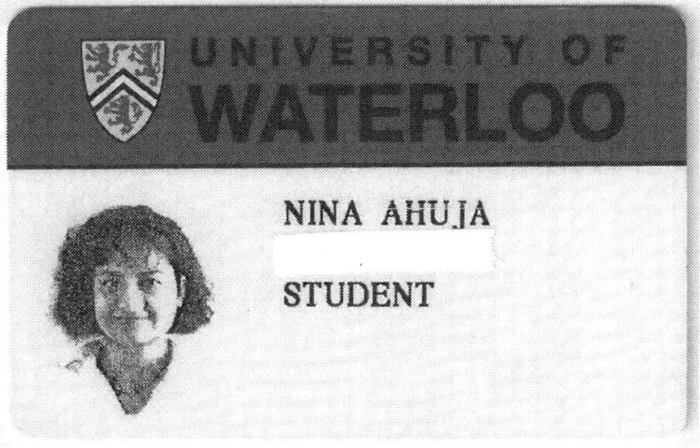

Now I decided to go for an even shorter and more layered hairstyle. That decision seemed reasonable to me at the time—new program, new look. Unfortunately, for someone with naturally curly hair, this was a bad decision.

Enter Exhibit B, a truly unfortunate photo.

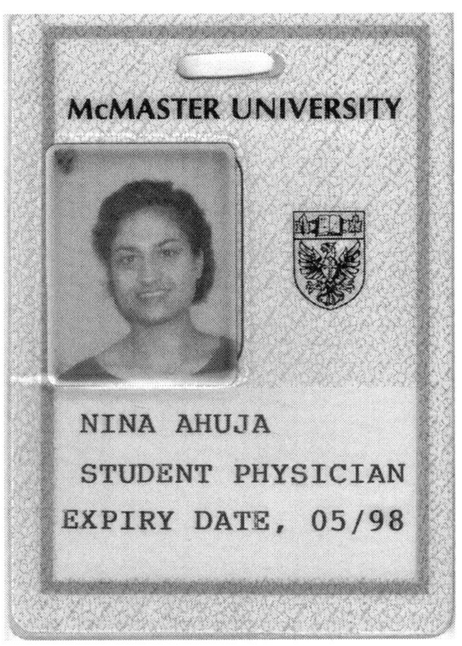

Starting medical school was an exciting time. It was also a period of uncertainty and anxiety. I frequently wondered: What was medical school really going to be like? Would I rise to each challenge, as I always had in the past? How would I manage the heavy weight of responsibility inherent to caring for others? Would I thrive? Would I enjoy it? Would I feel overwhelmed? Looking back on my various ID badges over the years, I have come to realize that my frequent response to these questions was to get my hair "trimmed" each time I felt anxious. Enter Exhibit C, an ID photo taken during a stressful time in residency with yet another short haircut.

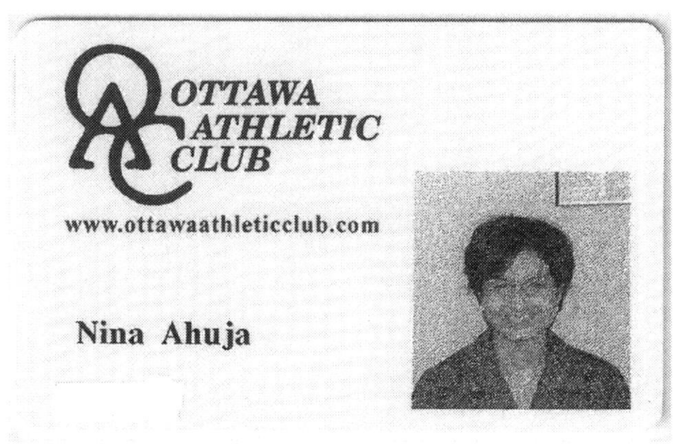

Before you learn how to manage stress effectively, you first need to understand your own responses to stress and how they manifest themselves in your world. Had I recognized back then that my impulse to have my hair cut was an indication that I was feeling overwhelmed and unsure, I may have developed different coping mechanisms that more actively supported productivity and worked better with naturally curly hair.

Stress can be both positive and negative. Positive stress is when you feel excited, without feelings of threat or fear. It can be motivating and help you meet your daily challenges with energy and enthusiasm. Reading your acceptance letter, starting a new program, performing your first procedure, starting your own practice—all these are experiences you may anticipate with positivity and that may inspire you into productivity.

Negative stress, on the other hand, can feel overwhelming and out of control. Multiple tasks with too little time, overwhelming volumes of work, and feeling completely disorganized. It is important to recognize how you experience stressful circumstances, so you can begin to manage your responses effectively.

STRESS, EMOTION, AND YOUR PERSONALITY

On an emotional level, stress may reveal itself as agitation, frustration, depression, a desire to isolate, feeling overwhelmed, alone, or even angry. Our reactions to stress, in turn, impact how we communicate and relate to those around us. As an example, in moments of acute stress I instinctively become quiet, emotionally withdrawn, and more formal in my tone and communication style. While my response does vary depending on the situation, it aligns with my tendency to be more introverted—going inward allows me to quietly reflect and objectively assess the situation at hand.

Personality traits impact how you respond to stress. Understanding your own tendencies is important.

Introverts tend to prefer time alone to restore their energy, think, and reflect. Excessive social interaction is draining for them, and while their friendships may be fewer in number, they tend to be close and deep in nature. When it comes to stress management, introverts have the advantage of greater self-awareness as they often take time to actively self-reflect. However, they also have a tendency to be less emotionally expressive and less willing to turn to others for support.

Extroverts, on the other hand, restore their energy by spending time with others and are happy to talk for hours. They thrive on social interaction and have many friends, though their relationships may not be as deep. When it comes to stress management, extroverts have the advantage of being willing to reach out to others for support and openly share their thoughts, fears, and insecurities. However, their tendency for self-expression can sometimes override their self-reflection, potentially limiting their opportunity for greater self-awareness.

While most people fall somewhere along the continuum of introversion and extroversion, there are helpful lessons to learn from both vantage points. It is important to recognize your own personality traits so you can seek support in stressful times, in ways that are not limited by your tendencies.

REFLECTION POINTS

- Would you consider yourself to be an introvert or an extrovert?
- Reflect on a time of acute stress in your life. Did you reach out to others for support or turn inwards?
- Considering your two responses, did your natural personality tendency help or hinder your ability to manage stress? If so, how?

OTHER STRESS REACTIONS

Stress can manifest itself in other forms as well. Besides the physiologic "fight or flight" response evoked in acutely stressful situations, physical manifestations of prolonged stress can include palpitations, chest pain, low energy, low libido, headache, and joint and muscle pains. Cognitive manifestations can be worry, forgetfulness, an inability to think clearly or concentrate, indecision, and general feelings of disorganization and pessimism. Then there are behavioral manifestations, like eating, sleeping, or working too little or too much, or relying on addictive substances or behaviors for relief and comfort. Some people have a tendency towards perfectionism, procrastinating, or completely avoiding issues. Still others exhibit nervous behaviors like fidgeting, nail-biting, or in my case, frequent haircutting.

Your response to stress is often proportional to the specific trigger evoking the response. There are relatively minor triggers like managing the unique personalities of our patients as we move from one examining room to the next, or constantly running behind in clinic and trying to play catch-up the entire day. Then there are the triggers that impact us more deeply and even personally. The overwhelming feeling from the sheer volume of work that needs to be done. The weight of knowing that every decision we make may have a major impact on a patient's life. The relief of patients recovering. The sadness of patients dying. The impact of how your colleagues or supervisors interact with you, amidst their own responses to stress.

From my days on rotation in cardiology as a first-year ophthalmology resident, memories of spending hours with a patient and his family in the emergency department stay with me to this day. Despite best efforts and multiple interventions through the night, the 82-year-old father, grandfather, and great-grandfather passed away silently with his family beside him. When the staff physician arrived on-site, he completed the death certificate and left without so much as a glance or word my way, despite my having discussed the case with him at multiple points through the night. No acknowledgement, discussion, case review, or other interaction. Only silence with the soft cries in the background of a family in mourning, and my heart heavy with sorrow. My supervisor's response and lack of interaction left me feeling alone, confused, and extremely upset. I had no idea how to process the experience, which added significant stress emotionally and intellectually.

All of these stressors are compounded by the nature of medical training itself: countless hours of clinical service with different supervisors on each rotation. The never-ending to-do list of preparing for clinical rounds and presentations, as well as studying for exams. The on-call assignments, research projects, and submissions for grants and publications. Then after you finish your training, your career becomes complicated in additional ways: managing the business aspects of medicine often with little to no formal training, and ensuring that legislated standards and practices are met in all aspects of your work. You continue to provide care to your patients and perhaps teach medical students and residents as well. And, at times, you put the health of your patients above your own, all while trying to balance family and personal life.

Chronic stress results from sustained activation of the acute stress response, which over time may lead to a state of emotional, physical, and mental exhaustion, otherwise known as burnout. Some doctors may feel they respond productively to excessive and prolonged stress, with a healthy diet, exercise, and other routines to help them cope. However, it is important for each of us to recognize when chronic stress becomes too much.

USING EMOTIONAL INTELLIGENCE

Consider for a moment the sequence of the acute stress

response in its simplest terms: emotional processing of a perceived threat triggers the hormonal cascade of "fight or flight" and the physiologic responses associated with it. Since emotional processing starts this sequence, learning to understand and manage our emotions is fundamental to managing stress, regardless of the trigger. This concept refers to "emotional intelligence," the ability to understand and manage your emotions effectively.

Based on measures of emotional and social competence developed by Reuven Bar-On,[*] there are fifteen inter-related competencies of emotional intelligence that impact psychological well-being. The three competencies primarily related to stress management are the following:[†]

1. Flexibility—your ability to modify your emotions and adapt to dynamic circumstances
2. Stress tolerance—your ability to manage challenging situations without developing physical or emotional symptoms

---

[*] Reuven Bar-On, "Emotional Quotient-Inventory," PsycTESTS Dataset, American Psychological Association (APA), May 7, 2012, https://doi.org/10.1037/t04985-000.

[†] Steven L. Stein and Howard E. Book, *The EQ Edge: Emotional Intelligence and Your Success,* 3rd ed. (Ontario: John Wiley and Sons Canada, 2011).

3. Optimism—your ability to maintain a positive attitude even in the face of adversity

As we move through the chapters and eventually work through the ADMIT framework, these three concepts will be revisited in various ways.

In the next chapter, we'll explore the root of stress: the nature of uncertainty.

KEY TAKEAWAYS

- Before you learn how to manage stress effectively, you first need to understand your own responses to stress and how they manifest themselves in your world.

- It is important to recognize if you are an introvert, an extrovert, or somewhere in between. This will help you decide how best to seek support in stressful times.

- Learning to understand and manage your emotions is fundamental to managing stress.

REFLECTION POINTS

- What are your emotional, physical, cognitive, and behavioral responses to stress?
- How would others describe your stress responses? Do your answers and theirs align?
- How competent do you feel in the emotional competencies relating to stress management: flexibility, stress tolerance, and optimism?

CHAPTER 3

═══

The Nature of Uncertainty

"The quality of your life is in direct proportion to the amount of uncertainty you can comfortably deal with."

—TONY ROBBINS

The *Cambridge English Dictionary* defines *uncertainty* as "a situation in which something is *not known*." In business English, the same dictionary defines *uncertainty* as "the *feeling* of not being sure what will happen in the future." Together, these definitions align with the truth that uncertainty is experienced at both intellectual and emotional levels.

When I was newly married and a third-year resident

in ophthalmology, I was diagnosed with rheumatoid arthritis. I had accidentally run over my foot with a stretcher a couple of months earlier, so I didn't think much of the minor discomfort on the side of my left foot until the day I was unable to walk. When I got out of bed one morning, my first step was met with excruciating pain. My fifth metatarsal head was hot and significantly swollen, so I immediately reached out to a former rheumatology supervisor, who was kind enough to assess me that day. When he first told me the diagnosis, I was in shock. I had no family history of the disease, and I was otherwise in perfect health. The erosions staring back at me on the X-rays were surreal. I couldn't believe what I was seeing and hearing.

From an intellectual perspective, my uncertainty around the illness itself was relatively low since I had studied the condition during my rheumatology rotation earlier in residency. From an emotional experience, however, I was overwhelmed with memories of patients with severe and chronic pain, as well as deformities in their hands and feet that limited their mobility and activity. These memories heightened the unpredictability of what would follow for me. Over the next year, as my condition progressed to both of my feet and then my ankles, wrists, and hands, everything I had worked so hard to achieve flashed before my eyes. How would this impact the remainder of my training? How about my career, marriage, and family? Would any of the available treatments work for me, and if so, for how long?

Just as the nature of stress varies from individual to individual, such is the case for uncertainty as well. Many people find it easier to manage the unknown from an intellectual standpoint. You can study an issue and lessen the uncertainty by assessing probabilities, based on what you have learned. However, it is tremendously challenging to manage the unknown from an emotional standpoint. Most people appreciate their routines and have their own habits and plans based on their expectations. Disruption and redirection to an unknown path can be uncomfortable and unwelcome, particularly if you feel like you have little control.

Perceived control, locus of control, and outlook are important concepts to consider as you evaluate how to manage your own responses to uncertainty.

CONTROL AND YOU

The more control you *believe* you have, the easier it is to manage the unknown. The very nature of uncertainty is the perceived lack of control, and the unpredictability associated with it. When you apply to medical school, residency, or a staff position at a new center, there are a host of uncertainties ahead of you: Will you be selected for the position of your choice? Where will you live? How will you transition? Will you make the right decisions along the way? In moments of crisis, the degree of uncertainty is even greater. Will you be able to make sense of the chaos around you? How will circumstances change? What unique challenges will come your way?

In uncertainty, then, with so many questions unanswered, how much control do you really have?

For individuals with an external locus of control, there is a sense that things happen *to* them due to chance or luck, with the belief that they have little control over the outcome. They tend to avoid the subject of uncertainty altogether. This has the short-term advantage of not having to confront the uncomfortable intellectual and emotional experiences that accompany the unknown. As time goes on, however, the disadvantages of this avoidance become more obvious. Situations continue to evolve while the issue continues to be avoided, with levels of complexity often increasing as time goes on. When people with this viewpoint emerge from their avoidance to finally deal with the situation, they often face even more unknowns: more unpredictability, more uncertainty, more increased risk, and even more stress.

In contrast, for people with an internal locus of control, there is a sense that success or resolution happens *because* of them, through their own efforts and abilities, and with the belief that they have significant control over the outcome. They actively confront circumstances around them and tend to view uncertainty as an opportunity to investigate, adapt, learn, and grow. While aspects of the unknown may remain unresolved, people with this viewpoint experience fewer feelings of unpredictability, risk, and associated stress. The emotional experience of uncertainty is more manageable and perhaps even productive.

Accepting uncertainty is a difficult thing. It challenges your ability to be open and flexible to circumstances that are constantly changing and in unpredictable ways. As a high achiever, you typically have a clear sense of direction on where you want to go and how you want to get there. There is often little willingness to waiver from this well-defined path, particularly if the alternative is uncertain.

IMAGINING ANOTHER WAY

Herein lies a challenge.

Imagine what it would be like to live in the present moment with only an overarching concept of your ultimate goal. You have no clear plan, no defined roadmap. Your focus is in the now, dealing with the situation directly in front of you. Each and every moment *after* now is its very own unique opportunity. The possibilities are endless, and as they present themselves, you will choose those that align with your goal. You have faith that you will be guided along the best path of discovery to take you to where you want to go. With your commitment and hard work, you will arrive at your destination with unexpected twists and turns along the way. It may not be how you thought it would be when you arrive, but the journey along the way helped you grow. Uncertainty paved the path for you to experience and evolve in a way that a path of knowing may not have allowed.

How does that feel?

Close your eyes and give yourself a moment to really imagine what it would be like.

Is it as though a weight gets lifted off your shoulders? Is there a lightness that initially feels difficult to internalize?

With repeated visualization, you can learn to shift your mindset and reframe how you experience the unknown. The word *opportunity* brings excitement and anticipation of what *could* come. With an optimistic outlook and reasonable degree of flexibility, stress associated with uncertainty can actually become a valued resource. It can offer a source of motivation for learning and exploring potential for new opportunities.

The stress response is intended to help resolve the perceived risk in uncertainty. A hormonal cascade heightens your senses and ability to respond to challenges. You become more alert, focussed, and more capable of processing and retaining information. This allows you to learn and be better prepared for similar instances in the future. For instance, the first time I was involved in a code blue as a final-year medical student on my internal medicine clerkship rotation, I was able to channel my initial panic into action. When the overhead page announced the code blue location, I began running towards the ward, all the while hoping I would *not* be the first to arrive. I had completed my advanced cardiovascular life-support training, but I had never experienced a code blue firsthand. When I entered the room, a senior resident had already taken the lead and asked me to assist with compressions. I didn't realize how much force each compression actually took and concentrated on putting my weight into each one. The heightened state of emergency and uncertainty turned into a heightened state of focus, and each skill I learned I would never forget.

Uncertainty is the root of all stress. By reframing uncertainty as opportunity, you build your capacity to manage unknown situations, increase your stress tolerance, and develop a constructive, productive, and positive relationship with uncertainty both emotionally and intellectually.

REFLECTION POINTS

- How much control do you believe you have over circumstances?
- Do you believe things happen *to* you or *because* of you?
- Do you approach things from a positive perspective, or is it your tendency to focus on the negative?

Understanding ADMIT

Now that we've explored the natures of stress and uncertainty, we can begin to talk about a way to evaluate where you are at and begin to meet the challenges you may be facing.

ADMIT is a framework that I created after recognizing that my own challenges could be organized into five phases of experience. It was born out of years of learning to manage my own stress in medical school, residency, and surgical practice; as an educator and leader in both academic and clinical institutions; and in my personal life. The framework outlines each phase of experience and common challenges to consider within each. As an acronym, the term is easy to remember. As a message, it encourages you to acknowledge and accept what you may be feeling.

In our physician culture of silence, the first step towards true wellness is to openly acknowledge and share our experiences, and to support one another without judgement. However, to be able to support one another, we must first be open and honest with ourselves.

To help you in this process, I share with you my ADMIT framework:

- Adapting
- Doing
- Measuring
- Introspection
- Transformation

Adapting presents challenges with changing your mindset to accept something new.

Doing considers our work as physicians, and the additional stressors beyond patient care.

Measuring speaks to the competitive culture within medicine, and how you define success.

Introspection emphasizes the importance of mindfulness and active reflection.

Transformation explores self-awareness and the impact that external influences have on how you evolve as a physician.

The following chapters will take a closer look at each phase of experience.

CHAPTER 4

Adapting to New Ways

"Change is the only constant in life. One's ability to adapt to those changes will determine your success in life."

—BENJAMIN FRANKLIN

Whether you are a medical student or resident, physician or surgeon, organization or system leader, new ways of doing things will always be on the horizon. Advancing technologies and virtual care are changing how we interact with our patients. Primary care health delivery systems are transitioning to more integrated models. COVID-19 abruptly changed how we all work and live, with new standards and social norms to maintain while continuing to provide the best care possible to our patients.

As with stress and uncertainty, we all experience change in our own unique ways. Adapting one's mindset to accept something new is the first phase of experience in the ADMIT framework. If you can adapt to a new idea or approach, your experience with change will often be relatively smooth. If you are unable to adapt to inevitable change, your experience will be much more turbulent and stressful.

When I first started medical school, I had a difficult time adapting to the learning style in my new program as I mentioned earlier. At the time, McMaster University's medical curriculum was almost fully self-directed and problem-based with very few didactic sessions covering core content. While I appreciated independent problem-based learning, I struggled with defining endpoints for myself when studying cases at hand. Coming from the more traditional style of didactic teaching, I was used to being provided with all of the necessary content there was to learn. There was comfort in knowing that if I diligently studied what had been provided, I could feel secure in my knowledge and confidently move forward. However, in this self-directed program, it was my own responsibility to compile and then learn the necessary content.

Even though the learning goals and objectives for each case were determined during our tutorial sessions within our small groups of four or five medical students, I found it difficult to set limits in the content-gathering process. My tendency towards perfectionism compelled me to go beyond what had been stated. My attempts to learn every possible permutation of each case began to work against me: I often felt overwhelmed with details. Even though my evaluations were overwhelmingly positive, I still found myself spiraling into a steady state of self-doubt.

Changing this mindset was a challenge. With fewer quantitative measures to gauge my progress, I had to adapt by establishing new accountability measures for myself to help me recognize what I had achieved. I set a certain number of study hours required each day and kept a log so I could track my progress. I purchased medical textbooks that presented content in a problem-based format, to help me learn and adapt to the new learning style. I learned to use traditional textbooks more effectively and to set limits on how far to go with respect to more detailed content. I developed a comprehensive study plan that met my needs and helped me emerge from self-doubt.

THE IMPORTANCE OF ASKING

Most often we go about our everyday routines without consciously realizing that things can be done differently. When new ideas or circumstances are presented—whether by choice or not—they can jolt us out of status quo and get us thinking:

> What is the purpose of the new idea or circumstance? How is it different than the everyday we are used to? Is there a benefit to the proposed change? Are there lessons to be learned? Will the change make us, or the circumstances around us, better?

The first step in **Adapting** is to start asking yourself these sorts of questions. This will help you determine your willingness to change your mindset and accept something new. As you contemplate your answers and consider the value of the idea, you may identify reasons for you to adapt. This is especially important in circumstances where you feel you have little choice but to change. If you are able to connect with even one meaningful reason, you are more likely to adapt successfully.

Your outlook is also an important factor. If you tend to be optimistic and view change as an opportunity, you may consider it more, and with an open mind. But if your outlook is pessimistic, you may focus on everything that could go wrong and miss the potential that may be before you. Some people are predisposed to being pessimistic by their genetics, personal history, external circumstances, and stress levels. To support a more positive outlook, surrounding yourself with positive people, journaling what you are grateful for each day, avoiding negative interactions and violent media as much as possible, and focussing more on possibilities instead of roadblocks you may or may not face along the way, all can be helpful.

The need to adapt can come in many forms. Sometimes it relates to the physical environment, like when your clinic moves to a new location. At times it relates to process, like determining your new office flow after implementing electronic medical records. Adapting can be at an intellectual level, like learning a new concept or skill. It can also be at an emotional level, like dealing with the stress associated with managing complex cases. When you are finding it difficult to adapt to a new idea or circumstance, it is often helpful to take into account the ultimate goal.

COMBINING APPROACHES

When doing this, I recommend that you combine the ADMIT framework with a method of goal-setting that is used in many organizations. The **SMART** method, coined by G. T. Doran, helps to ensure that the goals you choose to set are **S**pecific, **M**easurable, **A**chievable, **R**elevant, and **T**ime bound. With the two approaches combined, you have a comprehensive method for considering new ideas and their value. While ADMIT helps you consider the psychological elements, SMART gives you guidance for how to act.

To illustrate how ADMIT and SMART can be used together to help overcome challenges, consider the following ultimate goal: learning to feel comfortable with sharing your difficult experiences with others, despite the culture of silence within medicine.

Once top of your class amongst only a select few, in medicine you are now surrounded by a multitude of high achievers who have accomplished just as much as you have, if not more. You have all succeeded in highly competitive environments to get to where you are now. When you suddenly find yourself struggling and feeling overwhelmed in this world, you may feel hesitant to share with others for fear of being judged as weak or incapable in some way. Why is this the case? How can this be overcome? You can use the ADMIT framework to help identify challenges to conquer, with your ultimate goal in sight.

Here is where your contemplation begins.

In learning to feel comfortable with sharing difficult moments with colleagues, you may be struggling with any of the five phases of experience alone or in combination. Perhaps your *challenge* is **A**dapting to a non-competitive mindset, where your *goal* is to enjoy the company of excellence while still recognizing your own. Perhaps your *challenge* is in **D**oing—openly sharing your personal challenges, with the *goal* of being vulnerable with those you trust. Your *challenge* may be in **M**easuring your progress in developing relationships, with the *goal* of establishing meaningful social networks with colleagues. **I**ntrospection may be the *challenge* where you need time to reflect, with the *goal* of increasing awareness of your feelings and learning when it would be helpful for you to share. Your *challenge* may be **T**ransformation in allowing new ways to become part of your value system, with the *goal* of personal and professional growth.

After you have considered the phases of experiences in the **ADMIT** framework, your process of evaluating your willingness to adapt becomes clearer and leads to the following high-level questions:

1. If the intended goal or outcome is achieved for each phase, will your struggle be lessened in some way?
2. Will it be worth putting forth the effort to adapt and carry the process forward through to Transformation?

If the answers to both questions are yes, your mindset will allow you to accept the new idea and move onto preparing for change by setting SMART goals. These are based on the challenges and goals you identified as you worked through the ADMIT framework. As an example, for the more specific challenge of Adapting to a non-competitive mindset with the goal of enjoying the company of excellence while still recognizing your own, a SMART goal could look something like this:

- Specific: "To learn to appreciate my own progress while celebrating the success of others, by consciously recognizing my own achievements each day."

- **Measurable:** "1. In a personal journal, after 10 minutes of reflection, I will write down five examples of things I accomplished that day and felt good about, big or small, or did better than the day before. 2. I will take 10 minutes to speak with a colleague from work, to acknowledge and celebrate his or her accomplishments."

- **Achievable:** "1. I will schedule 20 minutes before bed, for self-reflection and journaling, at least twice per week, and I will review my entire journal before bed every Sunday night. 2. If I do not have the opportunity to speak with a colleague during the work week, I will call a colleague Saturday morning at 10 a.m. to catch up, share my goal, and invite them to share an accomplishment of their own, big or small, if they feel comfortable."

- **Relevant:** "I feel motivated to feel more united with my colleagues and to celebrate others' successes without feeling competitive."

- **Time bound:** "Three months, starting from this evening."

If the answer to both questions is no, however, given the choice, you may prefer to maintain status quo or consider an alternate option if any are available. Regardless of your answers, two additional factors come into play consciously or subconsciously—your source of motivation and your capacity for intellectual and emotional flexibility.

WHAT MOTIVATES YOU?

In the last chapter we explored the concepts of external and internal loci of control. When it comes to motivation, similarly, people are driven to do things for different reasons: extrinsically motivated individuals are driven more by tangible outcomes *outside* of their own inner experience, while intrinsically motivated individuals are driven by the *inner* experience of achievement.

Take, for instance, the following goals: earning your medical degree, earning a higher rank in faculty appointment, receiving an award recognizing your efforts, reducing wait times in clinic, and achieving lower complication rates for procedures. The *extrinsically* motivated person would feel driven by the objective outcomes of the achievements themselves— the degree, the promotion, the award, the reduction in wait time, the lowered complication rate—some of which could lead to additional external rewards like research opportunities or alternative sources of funding for expanding initiatives.

For the same goals, the *intrinsically* motivated person would be driven less by the objective markers and more by their inner experiences—increasing confidence and self-esteem, feeling satisfaction from progressing to their fullest potential, feeling better equipped to help others and bring about change in a socially responsible way. All of which can translate to improved relationships and increasing competencies, including clearly expressing ideas, making decisions, and managing stress.

For most of us, there are both external and internal motivating factors for everything we do. The more alignment between the goal and our values as a person, however, the more willing we are to adapt to new ways, even if our tendency is to be extrinsically motivated. Awareness of your values can be extremely beneficial for adapting, regardless of your primary source of motivation.

A NEW WAY

For the past 10 years, I have been caring for a remarkable 91-year-old patient who lives alone despite significant hearing impairment and severe bilateral vision loss, both acquired. She is an intelligent woman who typically has questions that are difficult to answer due to barriers in communication. When I first met her, she used a personal hearing amplifier that I would speak into slowly and loudly. My staff began booking her appointments first thing in the morning when there would be fewer patients in the office who might overhear our conversations. As time went on, her hearing impairment progressed, and unfortunately the personal amplifier no longer helped. She suggested I spell out the words letter by letter on the palm of her hand. I initially felt overwhelmed because my answers to her questions were long sentences, so I wasn't sure if the new approach would work. However, with the inner satisfaction I feel when helping others (intrinsic motivator) and the happiness I knew she would feel if I was able to communicate with her effectively (extrinsic motivator), I applied her suggestion. As I outlined each letter on the palm of her hand and she put words together to complete each sentence, my overwhelming feeling was replaced with joy when her face lit up as she understood what I was saying. With both external and internal motivators at play, our aligned goals were achieved, with each visit ending with a hug.

Flexibility is the ability to modify your thought patterns, emotions, and behaviors to accommodate changing circumstances around you. It allows you to *adapt* to new ideas. Flexibility is influenced by your outlook, your perceived value of the new idea, and your source of motivation. It is also reflected in how you react to an idea that was not implemented as expected. Take, for instance, the SMART goal outlined above. If you have no access to a pen, do you decide not to journal that night? Or do you dictate your five examples into your phone? If the colleague you were planning to call is out of town, do you call someone else instead? When you call a colleague and they choose not to share, do you feel discouraged or embarrassed with having shared your goal, or are you able to hold on to the value of your goal and maintain a positive outlook? Learning from obstacles and feeling comfortable with disappointment allows you to be more open and willing to try. In doing so in a way that is true and authentic, you may inspire others to do the same.

We explore this further as we move into the next phase of the ADMIT framework: **Doing.**

REFLECTION POINTS

- How open are you to new ideas?
- Do you consider yourself to be flexible or more resistant to change?
- What motivates you to accomplish your goals personally and professionally?

Doing the Work

"Think not of the amount to be accomplished, the difficulties to be overcome, or the end to be attained, but set earnestly at the little task at your elbow, letting that be sufficient for the day."

—SIR WILLIAM OSLER, MD

Medical school was one of the most challenging and lowest periods of my life. When I first learned that I had been accepted, I was thrilled and excited. I knew that I could meet my goal of helping people and their families improve their health, and I also knew that I would be challenged in ways that would hopefully bring out the best in me. But after a year and a half in medical school, my confidence was waning. My difficulty in setting limits for personal learning objectives threw me into a defeating spiral of self-doubt. I had been a successful high achiever most of my life, so these feelings of inadequacy were new to me. I found myself in a constant state of extreme stress and anxiety. When I would study, I found it difficult to concentrate, and the muscles in my neck would tighten up, making it feel difficult to swallow. Even though I knew the material I was presenting, it became challenging to clearly express my thoughts in group learning sessions and patient rounds. I found myself constantly questioning if I knew enough, if I was good enough, and if I belonged in medical school at all.

At the heart of medicine is the ongoing expectation to perform at the highest level and in the best interest of our patients. Earning admission into medical school is competitive. Moving on to the residency program of your choice is competitive. When you complete your education and progress to independent practice, each decision you make impacts patients personally and in their most vulnerable moments. Each step of the process is crucial: performing a reliable history and physical exam, interpreting these findings together with the results of diagnostic tests, engaging with patients to elicit the most helpful information, and putting it all together to formulate a solution and deliver the highest level of benefit to each individual patient. Every single interaction, every single day, counts—regardless of how overwhelmed, frustrated, or disconnected you may begin to feel along the way.

Interactions with patients can be challenging. On one busy day, assessing patients in clinic, answering pages from the emergency department while on-call, and writing emails in between cases in response to an urgent administrative issue, I walked into an examining room to assess my next patient. When I introduced myself, the 75-year-old man seated in the examining chair in front me said hello as well, and then asked about my ethnic origin. I opened the patient's chart to review my notes and shared that while I was born in Canada, my family was originally from India. It was a pleasant interaction until he responded, "I drive exactly the kind of car you people from your country would expect an old rich white man to drive."

I was stunned.

Speechless and unsure of how to respond, I immediately redirected the conversation to the assessment. I was able to emotionally disconnect to remain professional and calm through the remainder of the interaction, but deep within I felt disheartened by his ignorance. When I shared this experience with a colleague, an emergency physician of African heritage, at a health finance course later that month, I learned that he faced similar interactions. It was both infuriating and comforting to know I was not alone. Our common interest in understanding health systems created opportunities for conversation and formed a bridge that made it easier to share our experiences.

A WORLD OF CHALLENGES

Life in medicine is not easy. Whether you are a medical student, resident, physician, or surgeon in practice, your work is multi-dimensional and comes with significant consequences to the lives of your patients and their families. You will deal with a multitude of personalities every day, each with their own emotional needs and wants. Language barriers and limitations make examinations more difficult, particularly when patients feel unwell and are unable to cooperate. Despite your best efforts and the time you spend, there will inevitably be those who will be unhappy with your care—medical or surgical.

No matter how experienced or exceptional you may be,

complications will happen. Every case is different, and every patient responds differently and in ways that you cannot predict. This truth keeps me at my best. Before the nurse helps me gown and glove in preparation for surgery, I always review my notes on the nuances of the case at hand. I mentally prepare myself for possible challenges so that my mind will remain clear, focussed, and decisive throughout the surgery. I do this for each patient and for every case, even the time when my thoughts were interrupted by the 67-year-old patient who was lying on the operating table and announced, "You better not screw this up or I'll sue you." I had just gently laid the surgical drape in place and was about to start his surgery under conscious sedation. I took a deep breath, exhaled, and intentionally refocussed my thoughts to the task at hand. Surgery does not always go as planned, and sometimes can go wrong, despite your best efforts.

And so, the stress builds.

When patients feel dissatisfied or deal with longer healing times under your care, it is difficult not to feel partly responsible for what they are going through. Even when my patient has a challenging personality, or if the likelihood of recovering from their condition or undergoing successful surgery was extremely low to begin with, I always work with the intention of being able to help each patient and improve their quality of life as best as possible. While infrequent, I feel the same deep emotional impact each time I have an unexpected complication. From my first complication when I was learning the procedure as a resident, to the ones I have had in my expert hands thousands of cases and nearly 20 years later, I am hard on myself because I care. In my post-case analyses of complicated cases, intellectually I may know I did the best job possible. However, in the spirit of humility, humanity, and reflective uncertainty, I still ask myself—could I have possibly done anything more? I replay the case in my mind as I drive home while trying to preserve some emotional reserve for my family.

And so, the stress builds.

Many say physicians are a privileged group, that we are fortunate to have had the opportunity to go to school and achieve, to earn the money we do, and to live comfortably. In these same conversations, however, professional and personal struggles, sacrifices, resilience, and grit in our commitment to care for others are rarely acknowledged in any meaningful way. Instead we are represented as currency on political balance sheets with concerns for public opinion seemingly leading all decisions. Publicly funded health systems often devalue our work with every fee that gets cut, with every resource that gets restricted, with every demand for us to do more with less, over and over and over again. All the while counterparts in the private sector work in financial models with relatively less oversight since they are not funded by public money. The uncertainty that our best interests will be protected justly by the very systems we serve continues to build and becomes harder to shake.

When we talk about physician wellness, our innate culture of silence about professional and personal challenges works against us. Our work itself is extremely demanding, and always has high stakes for those we care for. External circumstances that impact our work carry uncertainties that add more stress. Constantly feeling targeted as the financial solutions to greater health system issues compounds our burden. Ideas for broader accountability that includes physicians *and patients* remain unheard, whereas mutually empowering frameworks may actually serve to improve our health system overall.

PROTECTING EACH OTHER

Unless medical students, residents, physicians, and surgeons share our challenges and experiences with fellow colleagues, support one another, and remain united in our voice, external factors will continue to diminish the value of the work we do, and in turn impact our wellness. A 2019 article in the *Canadian Medical Association Journal* notes that "suicide is an occupational hazard for physicians" and that it is "the only cause of mortality higher in physicians than in non-physicians." The article goes on to note that "increased suicidal ideation begins in medical school," and it says, "In a recent meta-analysis, the prevalence of suicidal ideation among medical students was 11.1%. In analyses subdivided by time, 7.4% of students reported suicidal ideation within the past 2 weeks, and 24.2% within the past year."[*]

Remaining silent will *not* help physician well-being. It will *not* help reduce physician overwork and burnout. It *will* perpetuate physician disconnection and poor mental health.

However, to speak your truth can be challenging. You

[*] Joy Albuquerque, and Sarah Tulk, "Physician Suicide," CMAJ 191, no. 18 (May 6, 2019): E505; DOI: https://doi.org/10.1503/cmaj.181687.

are amongst highly accomplished colleagues where sharing your most difficult and painful moments may bring fears of being judged as weak, incapable, difficult, or rebellious as examples, any or all in combination. The reality is that we all face significant challenges at one point or another—*we just don't talk about them.*

Why not?

We explore this idea more as we turn to the next phase in the ADMIT framework: **Measuring Success.**

KEY TAKEAWAYS

- Physicians face multiple sources of stress and uncertainty in the totality of the work we do.

- Despite the many challenges and external influencers that seem limited in their support of physicians, we remain steadfast in our commitment to providing excellent patient care always.

- Openly sharing our challenges is essential for well-being for ourselves, our families, our patients, and the health systems within which we work.

REFLECTION POINTS

- In your medical career so far, what experiences

have caused you significant stress professionally and personally?

- Did you share these stressful experiences openly with fellow colleagues?
- If so, did you allow yourself to be fully open and vulnerable? Why or why not?

CHAPTER 6

Measuring Success

"Whether you're being bombarded with problems, respon-sibilities, even insurmountable hurdles, when looked at as a test, you always have a chance to succeed, in the sense of rising above that which is challenging you."

—RICHARD CARLSON, PHD

Like many professions, medicine is inherently a competitive culture. You compete to earn admission into medical school, and then into a residency program of your choice. If you chose to pursue fellowship, you are competing for a position yet again, followed by jobs and hospital resources, depending on the nature and location of your practice. It is a constant state of comparing yourself with others to establish a competitive advantage for purposes of "winning"—how can you become a more ideal candidate? The expectation to perform at the highest level becomes part of how you think, whether you are preparing for a presentation or carrying on with your daily work. Excellence is always the expected standard.

In traditional methods of assessment, your capabilities and potential are measured using external measures of performance. This is what we are used to—grades on written and oral exams, the number of unassisted procedures we performed as a resident, our rate of complications, our evaluations from preceptors and peers, our number of research publications and presentations at conferences, our reference letters, our credentials and awards. External measures are important to help identify our strengths and weaknesses from an objective perspective, and to ensure that we have met certain standards and competencies. However, they are not the only measure of success and are arguably less impactful than the internal measures we set for ourselves.

During my final months of medical school, I had been preparing for the Licentiate of the Medical Council of Canada (LMCC) Part 1 exam, the first of two qualifiers that meet the Canadian Standard for independent medical practice. I had overcome difficulties during my medical education and felt confident that I would pass with flying colors. On the day of the exam, however, memories of my challenging journey in medical school triggered the self-defeating spiral I had fought so hard to conquer. My mindset became fixed in self-doubt and was difficult to escape in the moment. I failed the exam. I was devastated and felt like an imposter.

Compelled by my need to be fully transparent, within the first weeks of starting residency I met with my program director. I told him that I had failed my exam, and it may have been a mistake to select me for their program. I held my breath and awaited his reaction, unsure of what would happen next. To this day I vividly remember his response, delivered with kind eyes and a reassuring smile.

"Nina, everyone can have a bad day," he said. "And no, we did not make a mistake."

My fear of being kicked out of the program did not come true. My fear of being judged negatively and my news being held against me was instead met with supportive words, understanding, and compassion. After our conversation, I went to the nearest restroom and shed tears of emotional relief.

I successfully wrote my exam a year later. But the disappointment lingered with me for years. I rarely spoke openly of my initial failure. Part of my identity had been rooted in excellent achievement through most of my academic career. I had never failed to meet an external measure of success. Once I became surrounded by accomplished colleagues whose opinions I valued and respected, my awareness of their caliber made it difficult to share this particular vulnerability. I couldn't help but anticipate negative judgement—perhaps an unfair assumption projected onto others from the loudest critics of all: me, myself, and I.

YOUR INNER CRITIC

Internal measures of success are inherent to how you see yourself and what you believe you are capable of accomplishing. When your own expectation of performing well on an external measure is not met, your inner critic can be harsh and piercing. Your confidence and sense of self-security may gradually wane, and despite all other evidence to the contrary, you may begin to feel like an imposter waiting to be exposed.

Imposter syndrome is a common experience felt by many of us at one point or another. I certainly felt it. When I suddenly had difficulty when learning was once easy, I began to feel inadequate. When I needed to ask for help for the first time, I began to feel self-doubt. When I set the unrealistic expectation to be a medical expert yesterday even though I was in the first month of a new program, I constantly felt like I didn't know enough, and my feelings of self-doubt deepened.

By primarily focussing on external measures of performance, I had inadvertently set myself up for failure. Rather than *myself* recognizing and putting value on how hard I worked and how much I had progressed, my sense of achievement focussed on external reinforcement, an ironic mindset for me to have.

My parents always said, "So long as you work hard and put forth full effort honestly and sincerely, don't worry about the results—they will come naturally." Their emphasis was always on doing my best from an internally measured perspective. Somehow I had forgotten this, and in doing so I also forgot that challenges help me grow, that asking questions expand my understanding, and that not knowing everything is a necessary state of mind to remain humble and open to constructive criticism and new ideas. Instead I procrastinated to avoid feeling overwhelmed, judged myself from a hypercritical perspective, and worked extra hard to learn as much as I could to feel worthy of the positive opinion others may have had of me. It became a competitive state within myself that stemmed from an imbalanced emphasis on external measures of success, consciously or subconsciously, that in turn had an unhealthy impact on my inner sense of self and belief in what I was capable of doing.

While maintaining humility and being open to constructive feedback, learning to define yourself beyond the outward expectations of others is essential for developing a strong inner sense of self, for managing stress, and also for overcoming imposter syndrome. Fundamental to self-development is having a growth mindset where all circumstances, simple or challenging, are considered unique opportunities for learning. This perspective allows you to have a positive outlook and to work from an internal locus of control. You can manage the difficult clinical or surgical case, not because the nature of the case allows you to do so, but because you have the necessary knowledge, skills, and ability to deal with whatever challenges may come your way.

Your source of motivation is also impactful in developing your inner sense of self. Internal motivators support you as you strive to improve for your own satisfaction of accomplishing a goal, learning something new, or putting forth full effort towards something you believe in. Your greater objective becomes reaching your fullest potential with sincere effort, perseverance, and confidence in yourself regardless of the external measure of success.

Whether you are in medical school, residency, fellowship, or independent practice, you will always be judged by the world around you. External measures of success are objective indicators of your performance, the impact of which depends on the context, purpose, and value to those who are judging, both professionally and personally. More integral to your self-concept are the internal measures of success that you determine to be in alignment with your values, morals, and beliefs. Maintaining a flexible and growth-oriented mindset welcomes measures of success, both external and internal, and constructive feedback from others as well. Be honest, humble, authentic, kind, compassionate, and fair with yourself. Take time to be mindful and actively reflect from within.

This takes us to the next phase in the ADMIT framework: Introspection.

REFLECTION POINTS

- How competitive are you with yourself and with others?
- How do you respond when you succeed or fail?
- How do you measure your own success?

CHAPTER 7

Introspection

"The highest levels of performance come to people who are centered, intuitive, creative, and reflective—people who know to see a problem as an opportunity."

—DEEPAK CHOPRA, MD

Introspection is about examining your thoughts, emotions, and behaviors to understand how and why you react to things as you do. Central to this process is mindfulness, the state of being mentally calm and present in the moment. When your mind is calm and present, you can be more aware of any emotions or thoughts you may be experiencing. Then, with active reflection, you have an opportunity to explore your emotional state, its triggers, and in turn how best to manage your emotional responses.

We experience emotions in every situation—positive, negative, or somewhere in between. Take, for instance, Patient A, who is grateful for your care and engaged in pleasant conversation. You may feel happy for their comfort and recovery. You may recognize the feeling, and perhaps enjoy it for a moment, then move on to assess Patient B. Here you have a completely different encounter: Patient B didn't follow your previous recommendation for treatment, and repeatedly expresses the same complaint. You may feel annoyed and frustrated with the difficult conversation. You still provide the best care you can, and then move on to the next patient.

So far, you have internalized these interactions. Perhaps at some point you share these experiences with your colleagues. You express your joys and vent your frustrations, hear their experiences as well, and then continue with your usual routine. Sharing your experiences and describing events and emotions may help each of you relieve stress. It may also help you identify what impacts you personally.

With mindfulness and active reflection, introspection takes this a step further.

MINDFULNESS AND LISTENING

The concept of mindfulness is about paying attention
and being present in the moment. It is about clear-
ing your thoughts and being focussed, still, and quiet
enough to allow messages within you to rise to your
awareness. There are many ways to quiet your mind.
Many suggest focussing on your breathing. For me,
listening for the silence within the sounds around me
helps me feel centered fairly quickly. I then focus on
breathing deeply to help relax my mind and to allow
emotional or physical signals to come into my awareness. Creating space for my inner messages in this way
helps me identify disruptors of my well-being. It taps
into my intuition and inner sense of direction, allowing me to listen and later evaluate each message. By
doing so, I am able to understand myself more and
can develop ways to respond to emotional triggers
more effectively. This in turn helps me deal with negative thoughts and emotions and also helps manage
my stress.

THE POWER OF REFLECTION

After you become aware of your emotions and
acknowledge their presence, you move on to active
reflection. What I find most useful in this practice is

to ask myself questions from two perspectives—from my own, and also from the perspective of the trigger of my emotional response.

Consider the example of the two different patient experiences mentioned at the beginning of this chapter. From your perspective, actively reflecting on the emotional response to Patient A would involve asking questions about *why* you felt happiness in the moment. Did the interaction evoke your sense of empathy? Did it give you a feeling of personal satisfaction in having helped someone in need? Did you feel a sense of connection in the warmth of the interpersonal exchange? As for Patient B, your questions would be about *why* you felt irritated and frustrated in the moment. Did you feel like your expertise was dismissed when the patient didn't follow your recommendation? Did you feel like your patient was not engaged in your interaction? Did it seem like your time and those of other patients waiting to be seen was not valued and respected?

From the perspective of the trigger of your emotional response, you would ask yourself questions on how your own behaviors and emotions may have impacted the interactions with each patient: Did you listen to each patient differently—perhaps one with more empathy, and the other with concerns about time constraints? Did you explain your recommendations to each patient clearly, while preventing information overload? Were you equally receptive to hearing each patient's questions, or were you distracted by your own personal thoughts and concerns?

What lessons could you learn to help manage your emotional responses more effectively in similar circumstances in the future?

Herein lies the value of introspection. Through mindfulness and active reflection, we can develop greater understanding of the root of our emotions, how they present themselves, how they impact us and others, and how we can manage them most effectively. This is the essence of emotional intelligence, also referred to as emotional quotient (EQ).

EMOTIONAL INTELLIGENCE

My appreciation for frameworks of emotional intelligence came when I earned my certification as an EQ-i 2.0® Emotional Intelligence Assessment provider. Having worked with fellow physicians following their individual EQ assessments, and having been coached in follow-up to my own EQ assessment, I have come to realize that exploring emotions within a framework of competencies offers a structured and relatively organized way to gain deeper understanding of the complexities of your emotional self. The EQ-i 2.0® Model of Emotional Intelligence by Multi-Health Systems, for example, sets out five composite scales and fifteen subscales of emotional and social functioning that measure how well we perceive ourselves, express ourselves, develop and maintain relationships, effectively use our emotions to make decisions, and effectively use our emotions to manage stress. The EQ-i 2.0® is based on the original EQ-i authored by Reuven Bar-On previously mentioned in chapter 2.

COMPOSITE SCALE	SUBSCALES
Self-perception	Self-regard, Self-actualization, Self-awareness
Self-expression	Emotional expression, Assertiveness, Independence
Interpersonal	Interpersonal relationships, Empathy, Social responsibility
Decision making	Problem solving, Reality testing, Impulse control
Stress management	Flexibility, Stress tolerance, Optimism

From an emotional awareness and guidance standpoint, I am extremely blessed to have amazing parents who are always willing to listen without judgement and ask deeper questions with an unconditional love and acceptance that has never wavered. They nurtured my capacity to be mindful and actively reflect on my experiences and emotions as they happen. With that foundation and many years of life experience later, I continue to refine my skills in being introspective and realize its benefits more and more each day.

REFLECTING ON COMPLICATIONS

Nearly a decade ago, while in my eighth year of surgical practice, I participated in a medical mission in Bolivia that offered eye surgery to patients from remote areas. By then I was a well-established, comprehensive ophthalmologist and high-volume cataract surgeon with an excellent reputation in clinical work and surgery, as well as a lead surgical teacher for ophthalmology residents. Participating in a mission with like-minded colleagues was a wonderful opportunity to help those with limited access to ophthalmic surgical care. It was a meaningful experience that was in alignment with my goals and values of caring for others in need.

As expected in a remote area, surgical equipment and other resources were limited. This required me to use a modified technique for cataract surgery based on a method previously used in North America, and still routinely used in places around the world. While I was familiar with this surgical technique, I had little formal training in it and modified my usual technique to provide this care. I felt a tremendous sense of fulfillment after I operated on patients, no more so than when I removed surgical dressings the day after the surgery. Though language barriers often kept us from verbally communicating with each other, the patients' heartwarming smiles spoke volumes when they first realized they could see more than they saw the day before.

However, a few days into the mission, I had an unexpected surgical complication—an extensive suprachoroidal hemorrhage with no guarantee of vision recovery in the operated eye. While there had been pre-disposing medical conditions and other factors that increased the patient's risk, the complication impacted me profoundly. Immediately following the surgery, I went to the locker room, sat on a chair, and looked down to the floor, feeling completely disheartened. I forgot all of the successful procedures I had performed during this mission and could think only of this one complication. I began to feel my past self-doubts threaten to surface yet again.

By this stage in my career, however, I had honed a more mature and grounded mindset. I knew the level of expertise I had achieved through my career and was able to redirect my focus to the successful cases completed and the patients I was able to help. While feelings of disappointment and sadness about the complication stayed with me, I was able to return to the operating room and successfully complete my remaining procedures for the day.

Thinking back on this situation within a framework of emotional intelligence on a simplistic level for illustration purposes, my concern for the patient and my desire to help demonstrated empathy and social responsibility. Feeling discouraged, dismissing my strengths, and focussing primarily on the complication had struck my self-regard. Taking responsibility without acknowledging resource limitations and pre-disposing conditions showed inadequate acknowledgement of the reality of the situation. Recognizing feelings of self-doubt creeping up demonstrated emotional self-awareness. Returning to the operating room and successfully completing the day demonstrated optimism, stress tolerance, and flexibility.

Using an emotional competencies framework offers a concrete approach to considering the complexity of emotions you feel, and in turn helps you identify personal development goals you wish to achieve. In the above example, a number of insights were revealed that I could learn from. Increasing my emotional flexibility will offer allowances for when things don't go as planned. Acknowledging my emotions and strengths in difficult moments will help maintain self-awareness and self-regard. Assessing the reality of circumstances will help me be kind, fair, and compassionate towards myself. By enhancing these competencies, I can manage future emotional responses more effectively and manage my stress more effectively.

Introspection requires a level of honesty you may not feel comfortable with facing yourself, let alone sharing with others. But if you are willing to be authentic, difficult moments are learning opportunities that contribute to your growth professionally and personally. There are many ways we transform through life, both in external situations and from within.

Next, we'll explore this process further in the final phase of the ADMIT framework: Transformation.

KEY TAKEAWAYS

- Challenges and obstacles serve as learning opportunities for inner growth.

- Active reflection involves exploring your emotional responses to understand their origin and how they can be managed more effectively.

- Introspection helps develop emotional intelligence and enhances overall emotional and social functioning, including effectively managing stress.

- When you share your feelings with others, do you explore why you feel and respond the way you do?
- How often do you have the opportunity for mindfulness and active reflection?
- How connected do you feel to the root of your emotions and your ability to manage your responses effectively?

CHAPTER 8

===

Transformation

"A man found a cocoon of a butterfly. One day a small opening appeared. He sat and watched the butterfly for hours as it struggled to squeeze its body through the tiny hole. Then it stopped, as if it couldn't go further.

So the man decided to help the butterfly. He took a pair of scissors and snipped off the remaining bits of cocoon. The butterfly emerged easily but it had a swollen body and shriveled wings.

The man continued to watch it, expecting that at any minute the wings would enlarge and expand enough to support the body. Neither happened! In fact the butterfly spent the rest of its life crawling around. It was never able to fly.

What the man in his kindness and haste did not understand: the restricting cocoon and the struggle required by the butterfly to get through the opening was a way of forcing the fluid from the body into the wings so that it would be ready for flight once that was achieved.

Sometimes struggles are exactly what we need in our lives. Going through life with no obstacles would cripple us. We would not be as strong as we could have been and we would never fly."

—UNKNOWN

The broader concept of personal transformation is multi-dimensional and results in a new version of yourself each time you transform. As you move through life and its various phases of experience, there are periods of stability when you are living the life that you have created. Stable periods are followed by transition periods when decisions or circumstances drive you to a new way of being in one or more dimensions. This eventually circles back to stability, then again to transition, and so on.

Depending on how you engage within this process, your physical, emotional, cognitive, and behavioral responses can mold you in various ways. You may adapt to new ideas, accomplish unexpected goals, learn new ways of measuring success, and understand yourself more deeply. A positive outlook, a growth mindset, and introspection are all essential in helping you become a stronger and better version of yourself as you transform.

When I first entered medical school, the process of transforming into a physician began at the very outset. I was surrounded by peers who were pursuing the same profession with an inclusion that cultivated belonging. As I progressed through the curriculum and many new experiences, I achieved my goals with a passion to care for others. I could see the impact of my efforts in patients I managed, and their positive outcomes were meaningful and rewarding.

The challenges I faced helped me learn to give myself permission to make mistakes, to be kind when setting expectations for myself, and to maintain a mindset that was focussed on growth. On a practical level, I developed a habit of prioritizing and tracking my goals each day, making work feel more manageable and consistently productive. I learned relaxation techniques and consciously applied time management strategies to include opportunities for mindfulness and active reflection.

The overall process increased my mental toughness and ability to persevere.

Just like the butterfly, each obstacle helped me transform and made me stronger.

MAINTAINING BALANCE

Since the beginning of my journey in medicine, my philosophy has been to treat every patient how I would want my own family member to be treated, no matter what the circumstance, no matter how pleasant or unpleasant the patient. In more difficult moments, I manage the situation appropriately, and in a manner that remains calm and respectful. My approach holds true for all of my interactions and is rooted in the values with which I was raised. With the many influences that shape you—childhood upbringing, cultural upbringing, role models, and other social experiences—what roots you as you transform as a physician?

In answering this question, the concept of nature

versus nurture is an interesting consideration. While there is agreement that both genetic factors and environmental influences contribute to behavior and development, the relative contribution of each factor remains unclear. External influences are thought to enhance predisposed traits towards developing a superiority complex, for example, or an inferiority complex on the opposite extreme. In the high-pressure, high-stakes, and time-sensitive circumstances we routinely face in our profession, how do you maintain yourself in a healthy balance? How do you convey confidence and skill as a doctor, while maintaining a genuine sense of humility and compassion? And regardless of what your innate behaviour or personality tendency may be?

In the 1993 movie *Malice,* there is a famous scene where a surgeon (played by Alec Baldwin) is asked if he has a "God complex" by a prosecuting attorney (played by Peter Gallagher). Baldwin's surgeon character responds with the following monologue:

> "I have an MD from Harvard, I am board-certified in cardiothoracic medicine and trauma surgery, I have been awarded citations from seven different medical boards in New England, and I am never, ever sick at sea.

So I ask you: when someone goes into that Chapel and they fall on their knees and they pray to God that their wife doesn't miscarry, or that their daughter doesn't bleed to death, or that their mother doesn't suffer acute neural trauma from postoperative shock, who do you think they are praying to? Now go ahead and read your Bible, Dennis, and you go to your church, and, with any luck, you might win the annual raffle. But if you're looking for God, he was in operating room number two on November 17th, and he doesn't like to be second-guessed. You ask me if I have a God complex. Let me tell you: I am God."

This takes us back to the concept of emotional intelligence.

Consider Alec Baldwin's character within the emotional intelligence framework that was discussed in chapter 7. On a simplistic level for illustration purposes, the surgeon reflects high self-regard with low reality testing—he demonstrates an extremely high opinion of himself, does not appear to recognize his limitations, and rather sees himself as God, which of course, he is not. Also projected is a high level of assertiveness together with low empathy—he states his opinion clearly and without ambiguity, while not appearing to consider the thoughts and feelings of others, to the point of making him come across as aggressive, rather than assertive.

Emotional intelligence involves a dynamic set of competencies that influence one another and can evolve over time. If the surgeon wished to transform, the prior illustration reveals a number of questions for Baldwin's character to explore. What does the surgeon feel his strengths and weaknesses are, and is he willing to acknowledge and accept them? Does he believe in personal improvement and strive for meaning in his work *and* interactions? Does he recognize and understand his emotions and how they impact his thoughts and actions, and those of others? Does he keep the emotions of others in mind when he communicates his thoughts, wants, and needs? Does he strive to develop mutually respectful relationships characterized by kindness and trust? Does he remain objective and see things as they really are, or does he live in his own reality? If Baldwin's character were to explore these sorts of questions, he may enhance self-awareness and other competencies within the composite scales of self-perception and self-expression. This may enhance his interpersonal relationships, which in turn may support his ability to work with others, make mindful decisions, and manage stress more effectively.

Emotional intelligence is essential to understanding who you are and how you transform. This is especially important for us as physicians, since being a leader is inherent to our role.

As a highly educated health professional with unique skills and expertise, your central goal as doctor is to guide your patients to better health. With each successful medical or surgical intervention and each successful interaction, your position as a leader becomes reinforced by your patients, colleagues, students, and peers. Whether you are working in a clinic, managing your own private office, working within organizations, or teaching, you have a voice of experience to contribute that can benefit patients and health systems overall.

As an emotionally intelligent leader, you will have greater potential for impacting patients and our health system, and in positive ways that will extend well beyond your medical training.

Reflecting on your experiences and considering

them within the ADMIT framework can help you accomplish your goals. We are consistently **A**dapting to New Ways, **D**oing the Work, **M**easuring Success, being **I**ntrospective, and **T**ransforming in one way or another.

You can do this best when you have support systems to help you navigate your experiences and manage associated stress. We'll explore this more next.

KEY TAKEAWAYS

- Positive outlook, growth mindset, and introspection are all essential in transforming into stronger and better versions of yourself.

- As your identity transforms in any situation, your personal observations and external environment influence how you evolve as a physician.

- As a physician, you are inherently a leader. As an emotionally intelligent leader, you have the potential to impact in positive ways that will extend well beyond your medical training.

REFLECTION POINTS

- Reflecting on your career so far, how do you identify with your role as a physician? Has this changed through your medical career? If so, how?

- How have you transformed professionally and personally?
- What circumstances or events have contributed most to your transformations, and how?

PART 3

Support

If you reflect on your daily practice, how do you interact with your patients when you feel content and happy, versus when you feel frustrated or upset? How do you deal with the challenges of being a physician when you feel respected for your expertise and skills, versus when you feel like you are being treated unjustly? How do you deal with receiving an unexpected patient complaint, when you feel like you have provided the best care you can? How do you engage when you feel supported by those around you—your family, friends, colleagues, and systems—instead of when you feel as though you are in conflict?

I have come to appreciate the value of support in relieving stress from two perspectives: the emotional relief experienced from talking about concerns, and the opportunity created to see things differently. We all have our own interpretation of events that happen—our perceptions are often influenced by our past experiences, values, beliefs, and biases. Reaching out to others invites new perspectives to consider, which may change your perception and how you respond.

In stressful situations, the importance of supports cannot be understated. It can impact your outlook and how you evolve both personally and professionally.

CHAPTER 9

The Importance of Support

"Somehow we've come to equate success with not needing anyone. Many of us are willing to extend a helping hand, but we're very reluctant to reach out for help when we need it ourselves. It's as if we've divided the world into 'those who offer help' and 'those who need help.' The truth is that we are both."

—BRENÉ BROWN

The very nature of medicine is to provide care to *"those who need help."* As physicians we are amongst *"those who offer help,"* as a basic tenet of our profession. While doing so, we work extremely hard, often at the expense of ourselves and our families. How many times have you gone the first 10 hours of your workday without eating? How many nights have you slept only a few hours, if at all, because your work was so demanding? How many family dinners, children's activities, or recitals have you missed? How many weeks or months has it been since you and your partner spent quality time together?

While some choose to talk about their struggles openly, many stay silent and suffer in solitude. There is reluctance to share for fear of being judged negatively in some way, and for reasons we explored in chapter 5. This fear of vulnerability is not unique to medicine. However, in the context where our work significantly impacts patients' lives and excellence is always the standard, the tendency is to stay silent, especially when your highly accomplished peers seem to be managing quite well and rarely share challenges of their own.

When you choose not to share, dismissing challenges and the associated stresses can become a pattern of avoidance, as we explored in chapter 3. As you avoid these challenges, your stress will continue to build, as complexities continue to evolve in the interim. Over time, stress can manifest physically, emotionally, cognitively, or behaviorally.

Reaching out for support is therefore essential for maintaining your own health and well-being, both personally and professionally. Doing so, however, can be influenced by your personality tendency, as we explored in chapter 2. Introverts tend to be less emotionally expressive and therefore less likely to actively seek external support than extroverts.

When stress feels manageable and causes little disruption in your daily life, social supports such as friends, family, colleagues, and other social networks can be helpful in getting you through. When stress feels overwhelming and does begin to interfere, however, you may benefit from seeking professional support from a mental health provider.

As we explored in chapter 5, suicide is considered an occupational hazard for physicians.

I will never forget the moment when I learned that a longtime physician friend had taken his own life. My friend was younger than I, had been in practice for five years, and was married with a loving family. The last time I saw him, we shared funny stories, and he was excited to show me his new car. He appeared and sounded well. There was no indication that he was having a difficult time. Six months later, I was driving home after a long day in clinic when I received an urgent call from a mutual friend. I was shocked and in complete disbelief. My friend was a wonderful person, full of potential, with so much more to give to the world.

Stigma often discourages us from seeking professional help for mental health concerns. The stigma is often due to a lack of facts and understanding. In our world of medicine, however, we are introduced to mental illness as part of formal curriculum in our undergraduate medical education. We know the facts of these conditions, as well as the associated challenges they may bring.

Along with challenging our culture of silence within medicine, we must openly reject this stigma and be supportive of those who seek help. We should not be afraid to reach out to trusted relationships—family, friends, colleagues, mental or other health professionals—for the kindness, understanding, and social supports we need.

TYPES OF SOCIAL SUPPORTS

Social supports can be described in two broad and interrelated categories—types of support you may give and receive, and social integration where you feel connected with others through relationships. Valuable types of support you may give and receive include instrumental, which is more practical in nature; informational, which is related to guidance and advice; and emotional, which offers a safe space to express yourself without fear of judgement.

Instrumental support involves delegating tasks to those who are willing to help, so that you can be freed up for more pressing responsibilities. During residency, I made the wise decision to hire a cleaning lady to clean my apartment every two weeks. It was a form of instrumental support that addressed my more immediate and task-oriented needs. With the volume of studying that needed to be done and the long working hours as a resident, an untidy surrounding made me feel disorganized and would increase my levels of stress and anxiety. With the cleaning lady's help, I returned home to a freshly cleaned apartment and felt grateful and happy each time. I breathed a sigh of relief and felt light and energized. Instrumental support could also include asking a friend to run an errand or ordering takeout instead of cooking every meal.

Informational support is about seeking guidance, advice, tools, and resources to help deal with challenges. Senior medical students and residents, clinical and surgical supervisors, mentors and coaches, and family and friends can all offer valuable insights that may assist you in making thoughtful and well-informed decisions.

Emotional support is about sharing your experiences and feeling heard, understood, accepted, and valued. It is important to find people with whom you can share your innermost thoughts and feelings, knowing that they will be received with empathy, compassion, and no judgement.

My parents have been a source of unconditional support throughout my life. They provided a solid foundation for all I have been able to achieve. My elder brother shared perspectives based on his own experiences, and he also offered helpful advice I could always rely on.

I was also fortunate to have wonderful mentors

throughout my medical education. One especially played a pivotal role in my becoming the surgeon I am. From my earliest days in residency, he was always approachable and available to talk about cases, answer questions, share his own experiences, and offer advice. He was an excellent teacher and integral in helping me learn the techniques of cataract surgery. When I was diagnosed with rheumatoid arthritis, he offered both informational and emotional support, to help ensure that my residency training would be optimized as I learned to manage my condition. A role model who cared for patients with genuine kindness and concern, he often shared valuable life lessons I remember to this day, like when he said, "I've seen many docs get caught up in the world of fancy cars and big homes. It can create huge financial stress when you find that you've suddenly overextended yourself. Live well and enjoy your life, but live well within your means. Most importantly, avoid the mindset of 'keeping up with the Joneses.'"

Good mentors share their knowledge, skills, and advice, typically in a long-term association based on mutual trust and respect. In addition to offering guidance with their experience and expertise, they are also helpful in tracking development of professional competencies, identifying knowledge gaps, and helping the mentee create a personal learning plan.

If you have the financial resources to do so, consider hiring a coach, which is a shorter-term association with a more structured approach. Typically, a coach provides tools and assessment methods to help you identify your own goals and develop action plans to achieve them. For example, a coach may suggest an emotional intelligence self-assessment to help you identify your competencies and develop achievable action plans to help enhance them further. It may feel less emotionally vulnerable than sharing with a mentor.

Trust is absolutely essential when reaching out and seeking support from others. Trust is a feeling of safety that develops over time through consistency in attention, intentions, and actions. Do you feel confident that those willing to offer support will listen to you openly and without judgement? Do they provide the safe space you need to express your thoughts, emotions, and needs openly and freely? Do you trust that any guidance or help they may offer is ethical and in the best interest of your well-being? And in the spirit of reciprocity within social supports, can others trust you to offer the same patient ear, safe space, guidance, or help when they turn to you?

SOCIALLY INTEGRATED SUPPORT

About seven years ago I was referred a patient with severe autism who lived at home with his parents. He had an advanced cataract in his only functioning eye and had been assessed previously by three different surgeons, who all felt the surgery would be too risky. His devoted parents were desperate to help their son as they noticed significant deterioration in overall functioning as his sight worsened. Having heard about my work, the parents requested an assessment from me. The patient was so combative that I could not approach him long enough to perform a proper ocular exam. However, observing from a safe distance, I saw he had an obvious white pupillary reflex in his right eye that was consistent with an advanced cataract. I knew that to perform the necessary cataract surgery, the patient would require general anesthesia and all pre- and post-operative examinations would be limited. After extensive discussion of the risks and benefits, the parents understood the significant risks and consented to the surgery. With the help of my office administrative staff and ophthalmic technician, as well as the nurses, anesthetists, and fellow health professionals at the hospital, I was able to perform the procedure successfully despite a high-risk cataract with atypical features that required improvised techniques to complete.

At his post-operative visit in my office two weeks later, I was pleasantly surprised when the patient tentatively reached out his hand to shake mine. As I slowly and gently accepted his invitation, his grateful parents shared that their son had been calmer and was able to navigate about their home once again. A socially integrated network of support had made this happen. Everyone's contribution made a significant difference.

Social integration encourages connections that help you support one another in various ways. Other examples of socially integrated supports may include: Your cohort of peers in medical school and residency. Your circle of family and friends. Your peers in your faith group. Your fellow members in a club. If you can be open within these networks, share your joys and challenges, and listen and encourage one another as well, these interpersonal relationships can help you feel belonging and a sense of togetherness, which in turn will help you manage your stress.

While types of social supports and social integration are often discussed as concepts when exploring support for individuals, the principles also apply to organizations. Health and wellness programs are becoming more common in academic institutions and hospitals; however, organizational structures and processes also have a significant impact when it comes to stress.

Through most of my career, in addition to my surgical practice, I have been engaged in various leadership roles in both hospital and academic institutions. There are added responsibilities associated with these roles; however, I enjoy the variety of work and the opportunity to understand the world of medicine at broader levels. The associated stress is a form of good stress that has kept me motivated by being involved.

In one of my roles, however, I was impacted by a situation that generated a significant amount of negative stress. An ineffective reporting structure and pattern of mismanagement at senior levels enabled behaviors that were counterproductive. This significantly impacted team morale and my ability to fulfill my own responsibilities as a senior leader in a related role. My attempts to engage collaboratively to resolve issues did not work because the leaders responsible for managing the situation weren't motivated to resolve the challenges. It was an extremely stressful, frustrating, and demoralizing situation that rippled unnecessary negativity at multiple levels.

For a physician within any system, there is value in knowing that you can rely on your organization to effectively implement processes that support functional team dynamics. There is value in knowing that support will be provided appropriately should the need arise, and that you are recognized and appreciated as a valued member. For those physicians who enter leadership roles, being provided with essential training that is supported by the organization is powerful. Many physician leaders enter their roles with little formal exposure to effective management principles or legislative and regulatory standards. By expanding your knowledge and competencies beyond the silo of medical expertise, you will feel more empowered, more effective, and less stressed as you contribute to your organization. When systems succeed in providing supports and opportunities for you to be actively engaged and develop essential skills, your level of trust, commitment, and optimism builds. Failing to provide these conditions, however, feels disempowering and dismissive, erodes trust, and in turn further increases stress levels.

Just as in life, highs and lows in medicine are expected in all contexts associated with the profession. The importance of having social supports to help manage your stress effectively cannot be overstated. In socially integrated support systems, you can support one another in meaningful ways. Applying these concepts in organizations and systems can also be empowering and constructive.

Feeling heard and supported builds interpersonal relationships, which ultimately helps you manage stress. Be willing to share with trusted colleagues who understand the unique world of medicine.

KEY TAKEAWAYS

☿ Reaching out for support to help manage stress is essential for maintaining health and well-being.

☿ Social supports are described in two interrelated categories: types of support—instrumental, informational, and emotional—and social integration where you feel connected with others.

☿ To feel comfortable with reaching out and in turn seeking support, the element of trust is absolutely essential.

REFLECTION POINTS

- What types of social supports are available around you? How can these be utilized to help relieve stress?
- What social integration supports are available? How can you offer support to one another?
- Are there barriers for you to overcome to seek professional or social supports if you need them? If so, what are they, and how can you overcome them?

Conclusion

When I think about my journey through medicine, two things come to the forefront of my mind. The first is the joy of working with patients and helping them in their time of need. The second is the comradery I feel with my colleagues—my fellow physicians and surgeons, nurses, fellow health professionals, and support staff I have the privilege of working with each day.

It is important to reach out to each other, to connect, and to remember that we all share a unique bond and understanding in our world of medicine, with a shared history and experience that is both gruelling at times and also very rewarding. Reaching out and reminding yourself of this can be both comforting and helpful, especially in challenging times.

Stress in medicine is inevitable. With every challenge, we experience physical, emotional, and intellectual highs and lows. What I find to be most valuable is a positive outlook, flexibility, and maintaining a growth mindset—viewing each challenge as an opportunity to improve and learn.

The more connection and sense of alignment I have felt with my personal values and goals, the easier it has become to manage stressful moments. Drawing on elements of intrinsic motivation, internal locus of control, and other aspects discussed in this book, I created the ADMIT framework to help me conquer my own challenging moments. Considering the five phases of experience helps me identify sources of stress and, in turn, manage them more effectively.

As you navigate your own journey and face your own challenges along the way, my ADMIT framework offers an approach on how to assess your stressful experiences. It may help you develop an emotional self-awareness that will offer benefits both personally and professionally.

Here are a few final takeaways for you to consider that I have learned from my own mentors and experiences over the years:

1. Where there is a problem, there is always a solution. You just have to be patient and willing to look for it.
2. Where there is failure, there is opportunity for learning. Be open to reflecting on what lessons can be learned both personally and professionally.
3. Where there is conflict, reflect on intentions. If intentions are true and communication is mutually respectful, you will always find a road to resolution.
4. Where there is a feeling of lack of control, knowledge is powerful.

I wrote this book to share lessons I learned at various stages in my career when things were especially stressful. If this work can help even one person know that they are not alone in their journey, this book will have accomplished its goal.

I encourage you to challenge the culture of silence within medicine and wish you good health and wellness.

About the Author

DR. NINA AHUJA, BScHons, MD, FRCSC, CHE, is an ophthalmic surgeon and the Founder of Docs in Leadership.

After completing her medical degree at McMaster University, followed by residency training in ophthalmology at the University of Ottawa, Dr. Ahuja began her private surgical practice in 2003 in Hamilton, Ontario. As medical staff at St. Joseph's Healthcare Hamilton and faculty member in the McMaster Department of Surgery, she has earned numerous awards over the years for excellence in teaching cataract surgery, in patient care, and for contributions to medical education. She is currently Associate Clinical Professor, Academic Division Head for Ophthalmology, and an examiner for the Royal College of Physicians and Surgeons of Canada.

A Certified Health Executive with the Canadian College of Health Leaders, Dr. Ahuja has held numerous executive clinical leadership roles including Medical Staff Association President, member of the Medical Advisory Committee, and member of the Joint Board of Governors at St. Joseph's Healthcare Hamilton. She is presently a member of the Board of Directors at St. Joseph's Healthcare Foundation.

Drawing from her experiences as a frontline healthcare provider, private practice owner, and physician leader in both academic and healthcare institutions, Dr. Ahuja founded Docs in Leadership to promote and deliver physician-developed leadership curriculum for all health professionals relevant to the health system context. She is highly committed to ongoing personal and professional development and is certified in EQ-i 2.0® Emotional Intelligence Assessment.

Made in the USA
Columbia, SC
22 January 2021